CARDAMOM

MARIAN KIM

CONTENTS

MARIAN KIM

1

PROPERTIES

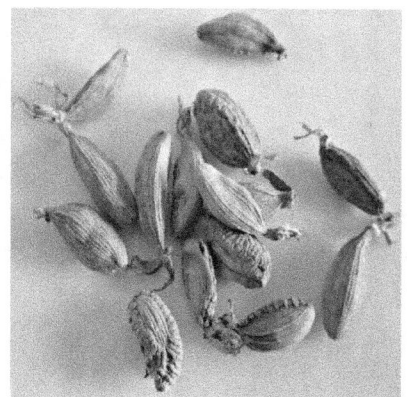

Scientific name: Elletaria cardamomum

Other names: Ela, cardamome

Properties

The properties of cardamom include:

Antioxidant properties

Anti-inflammatory properties

Anti-aging properties

Anti-cancer properties

Anti-spasmodic properties

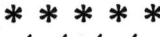

2

USES

High blood pressure treatment

Cardamom was shown to lower blood pressure in a study that was published in the Indian Journal of Biochemistry and Biophysics. In this study, participants with hypertension were given 3 gram of cardamom powder and noted to have lower blood pressure. Cardamom helps lower high blood pressure since it has diuretic properties.

Blood clot breakdown

The above study also found that cardamom broke down blood clots in the body. It also prevents the formation of blood clots which can cause strokes and heart attacks by preventing platelet aggregation and the sticking of platelets to artery walls.

Weight loss

Cardamom boosts the body's metabolism and enables it to burn more fat by virtue of being a thermogenic spice. This means that it increases the process of thermogenesis in which the body produces heat and burns calories in the process of doing so.

Cancer prevention

Cardamom contains indole 3 carbinol (IC3) and diindolylmethane (DIM) which are phytochemicals that fight hormone dependent cancers like breast cancer, ovarian cancer and prostrate cancer. Some research suggests that regular consumption of cardamom can prevent these cancers.

Digestive problems treatment

Cardamom is a carminative (digestive aid) and it is used to treat digestive problems like heartburn, nausea, acidity and intestinal gas as well as liver and gall bladder problems. Cardamom is also used to relieve stomach and intestinal spasms since it has anti-spasmodic properties. Cardamom seeds are usually chewed to relieve the digestive problems though the tea can also be drunk for the same effect.

Irritable bowel syndrome (IBS) management

Cardamom is used to reduce the symptoms of IBS.

Constipation treatment

Cardamom is used to treat constipation.

Anorexia treatment

Cardamom is used to treat anorexia or loss of appetite since it acts as an appetite stimulant.

Urinary problems management

Cardamom is used to relieve urinary problems since it has diuretic properties. These problems include burning or painful urination and frequent urges to urinate. It also helps in the passing of kidney stones.

Coughs and colds relief

Cardamom is used to relieve the symptoms of the common cold, coughs and bronchitis.

Sore throat relief

Cardamom is used to relieve sore throats and hoarse voices.

Halitosis relief

Cardamom pods are chewed to get rid of halitosis or bad breath after meals or whenever one needs to freshen the breath.

Mouth ulcers treatment

Cardamom is used to treat mouth ulcers, infections of the gum and tooth decay. Its anti-inflammatory properties also help reduce the pain and swelling in these infections.

Hiccup relief

Cardamom is used to relieve hiccups since it has anti-spasmodic properties.

Aphrodisiac

Cardamom is used as an aphrodisiac to manage erectile dysfunction and impotence.

Depression management

Cardamom tea is used to help fight depression.

Antiaging

Cardamom is an antioxidant which mops up the free radicals that damage cells and helps in resisting cellular aging.

Scorpion stings

Cardamon is used on scorpion stings.

Detoxification

Cardamom is used for detoxification since it helps the body expel wastes through the kidneys. It is also used for urinary problems since it acts as a diuretic.

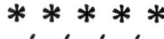

3

SAFETY PRECAUTIONS

Persons with gallstones should not use cardamom in amounts that are larger than those found in food since it can trigger gallstone colic.

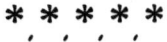

4

DRUG INTERACTIONS

None noted todate.

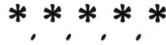

5

COOKING TIPS

Flavor: Sweetly spicy

Goes well with: Cakes e.g. coffee cake, cookies, spicy teas, fruit salad dressings

Can be substituted with: Ginger or cinnamon

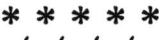

6

HERBAL RECIPES

Cardamom Decoction

Equipment

Non-reactive heavy saucepan

***

Ingredients

2 teaspoons cardamom seeds

1 cup water

***

Instructions

1. Place the cardamom and water in the saucepan, cover it and slowly bring the mixture to a simmering boil for 15 minutes.

2. Remove from the heat source and let the mixture cool to drinking temperature.

3. Strain the mixture, measure it and pour the liquid into a clean saucepan.

4. Heat the liquid until it begins to steam. Reduce the heat and let the liquid continue to steam until it is reduced to half its original volume. This may take 45 minutes to 1 hour.

5. Pour the decoction into a clean bottle.

*

Tips

1. Store the decoction in the refrigerator to lengthen its life.

***

Cardamom Tincture

Equipment

Glass jar with tight fitting lid

Dark tincture bottles

Cheesecloth

Labels

***

Ingredients

7 oz (200 gm) of cardamom seeds

30 oz (1 liter) of 80-100 proof vodka

***

Instructions

1. Fill 1/3 of the glass jar with the chopped herbs.

2. Add the vodka to completely fill the jar to the top.

3. Seal the jar and label it with the date of preparation and name of herb used.

4. Store the glass jar in a dark place for 6 weeks ensuring that you shake them weekly.

5. After 6 weeks strain out the herbs with a cheesecloth and pour the tincture into dark tincture bottles.

6. Label the tincture bottles with the date and name of herb used.

7. Store your herbal tinctures away from light and heat.

***

Tips

1. Pick your herbs early in the morning just after the dew has dried.

2. You can leave the herbs in the alcohol for up to 6 months if you want to create very strong tinctures.

3. To make your tinctures doubly strong, you can pour the tincture after straining in step 5 above and store it for six more weeks.

4. Though the dose varies, a standard dose is 1 teaspoon diluted in water or tea and taken 1-3 times a day.

*****

Cardamom Infused Oil

Equipment

Double boiler

Large glass bowl

Sieve and cheesecloth

Sterilized dark jars

***

Ingredients

16 fl oz. (500 ml) pure vegetable oil such as sweet almond oil or sunflower oil

8 oz. (250 grams) cardamom seeds

***

Instructions

1. Place the cardamom and oil in the glass bowl ensuring that the oil covers the herbs. Simmer them in a double boiler for one hour at a temperature of around 120 degrees Fahrenheit (49 degrees Celsius). Do not let the oil and herbs boil. You can repeat this step several times after letting the oils cool to create more concentrated herb infused oils. You can make your oils even more concentrated by adding a fresh bunch of herbs with each re-simmering.

2. Strain the mixture through the sieve and cheesecloth into a clean, dark jar ensuring you squeeze out as much oil as you can from the herbs in the cheesecloth.

3. Label your jars with the manufacturing date, expiry date, herb and oils used.

4. Store your herb infused oils in a cool dark place or in the refrigerator and use them within 3 months.

CARDAMOM

*****

Cardamom Salve

Equipment

Double boiler

Large glass bowl

Sterilized dark jars or tins

***

Ingredients

8 oz. (250 ml or 1 cup) herb infused vegetable oil (see previous recipe)

1 oz. (30 grams) beeswax

50 drops (2.5 ml or ½ teaspoon) essential oils like lavender essential oil

***

Instructions

1. Place the beeswax and herb infused oil in the glass bowl and melt them in a double boiler.

2. Once melted remove from the heat source and add the essential oils drop by drop until you get your preferred scent.

3. Pour the melted oils into the storage jars or tins and allow to cool completely.

4. Store the salves in a cool dark place.

***

Tip

If you want softer salves you can use less beeswax – for example ¾ oz of beeswax for 1 cup of vegetable oils.

*****

Cardamom Butter

Equipment

Large glass bowl

Electric mixer or stick blender or wire whisk

Molds such as ice cube trays (optional)

***

Ingredients

½ cup butter

2 tablespoons of finely crushed cardamom seeds

***

Instructions

1. Place the butter in a warm place so that it can soften.

2. Put butter and cardamom in a large glass bowl and blend well until thoroughly mixed.

3. Refrigerate until it hardens. You can refrigerate it in molds or ice cube trays to give it a special shape.

*****

Cardamom Tea

Equipment

Kettle

Tea cup

***

Ingredients

1 teaspoon of cardamom seeds

1 cup of boiling water

Honey to taste (optional)

***

Instructions

1. Boil the water

2. Put the cardamom in a tea cup, add the boiling water and let it steep while covered for 20 minutes.

3. Add honey to suit your taste before drinking.

###

ABOUT THE AUTHOR

Marian Kim is an experienced alternative medicine practitioner.

*****

OTHER BOOKS BY THE AUTHOR

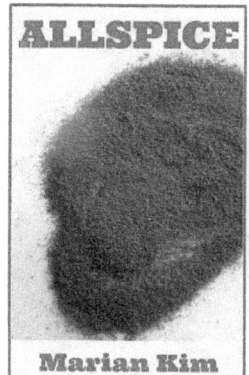

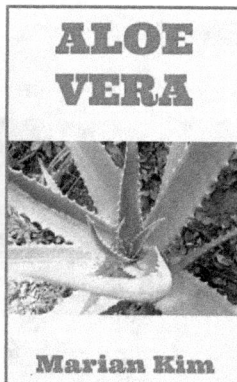

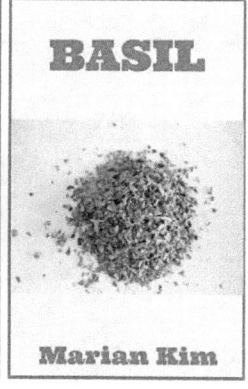

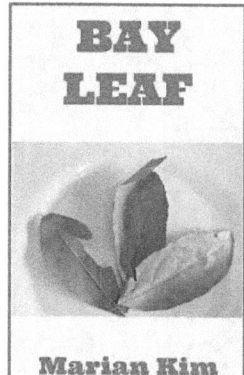

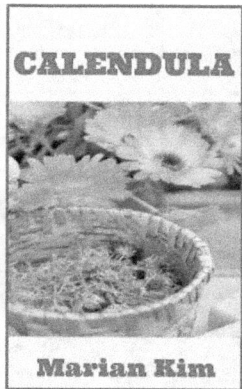

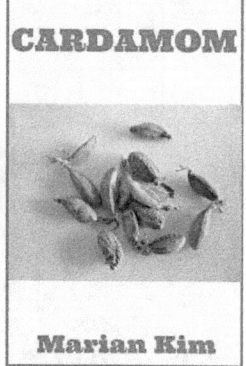

CAYENNE PEPPER

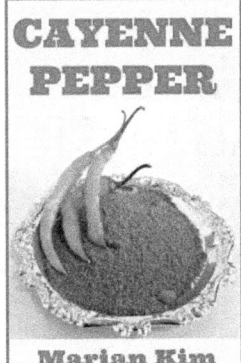

Marian Kim

CHAMOMILE

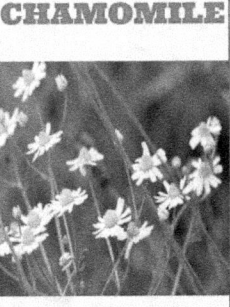

Marian Kim

CILANTRO & CORIANDER

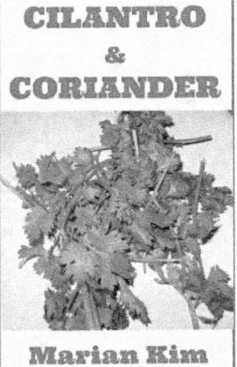

Marian Kim

CINNAMON

Marian Kim

CLOVES

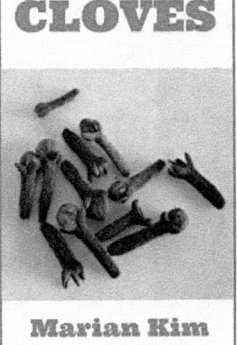

Marian Kim

CUMIN

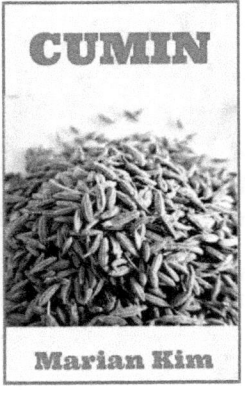

Marian Kim

DANDELION

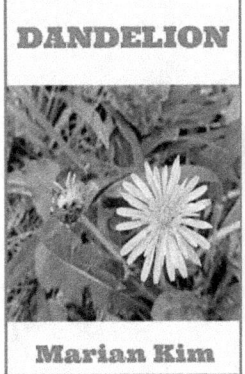

Marian Kim

DILL

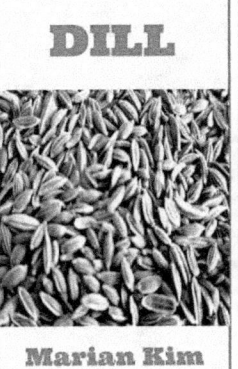

Marian Kim

ECHINACEA

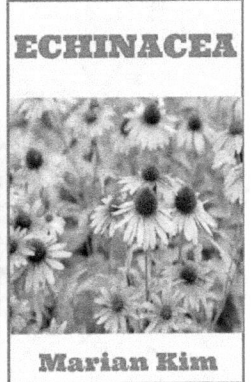

Marian Kim

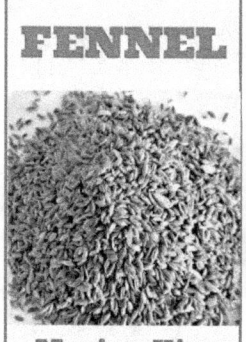

FENNEL

Marian Kim

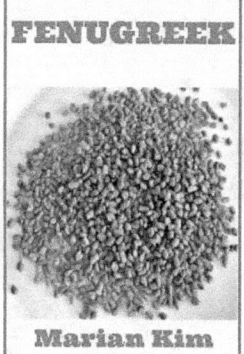

FENUGREEK

Marian Kim

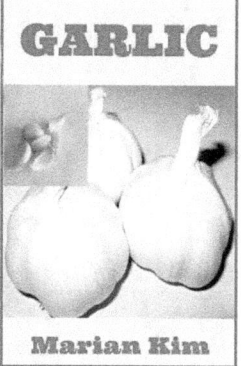

GARLIC

Marian Kim

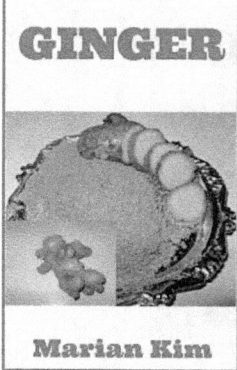

GINGER

Marian Kim

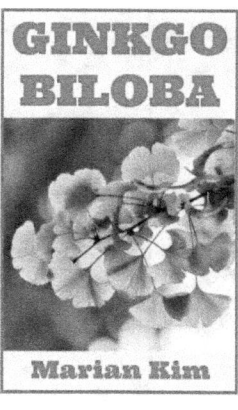

GINKGO BILOBA

Marian Kim

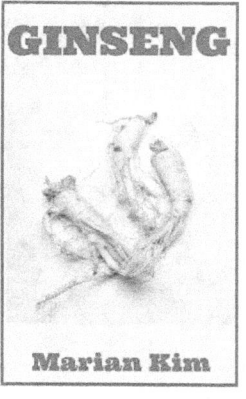

GINSENG

Marian Kim

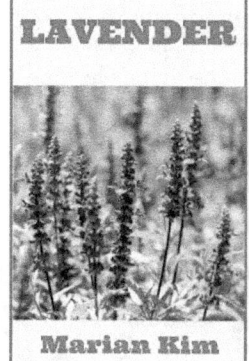

LAVENDER

Marian Kim

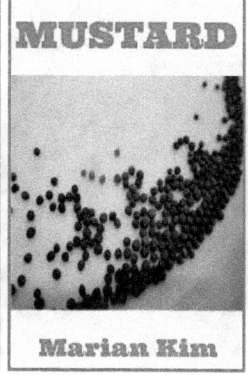

MUSTARD

Marian Kim

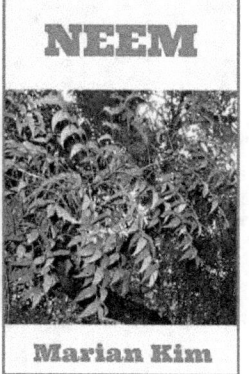

NEEM

Marian Kim

NUTMEG & MACE

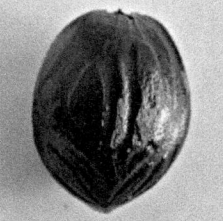

Marian Kim

OREGANO

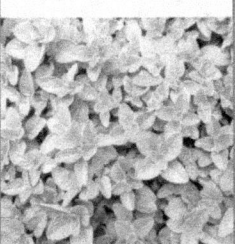

Marian Kim

PAPRIKA

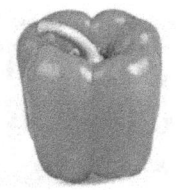

Marian Kim

PARSLEY

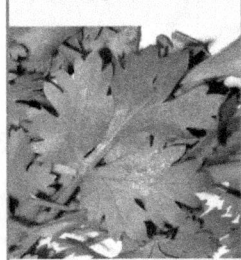

Marian Kim

BLACK & WHITE PEPPER

Marian Kim

PEPPERMINT

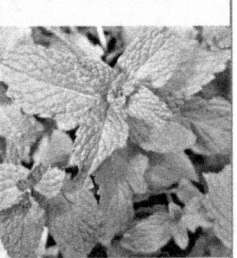

Marian Kim

ROSE HIPS

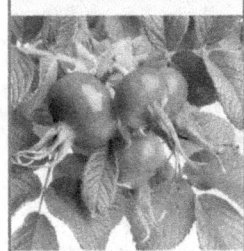

Marian Kim

ROSE PETALS

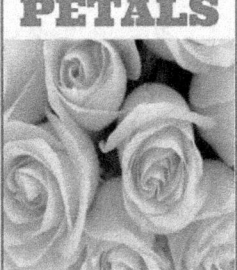

Marian Kim

ROSEMARY

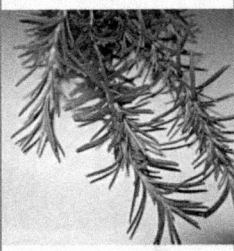

Marian Kim

24

SAGE

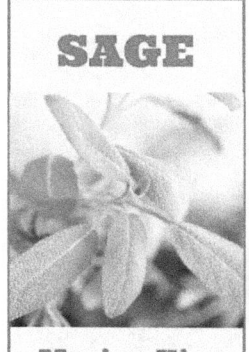

Marian Kim

ST. JOHN'S WORT

Marian Kim

STAR ANISE

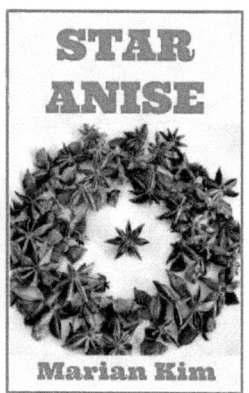

Marian Kim

STINGING NETTLE

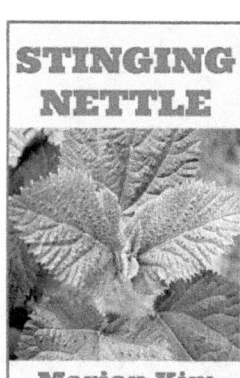

Marian Kim

THYME

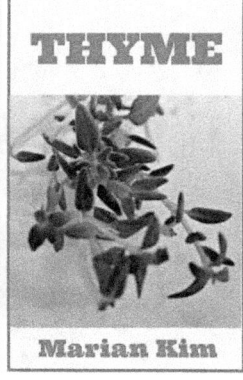

Marian Kim

TURMERIC

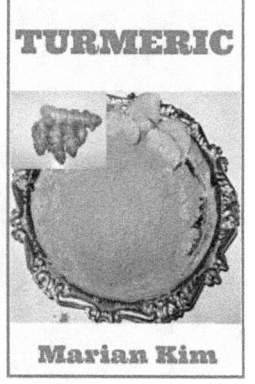

Marian Kim

WITCH HAZEL

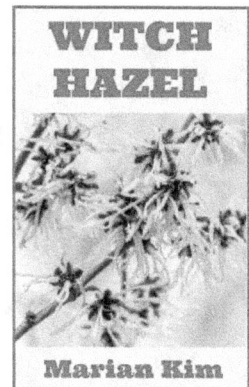

Marian Kim

YARROW

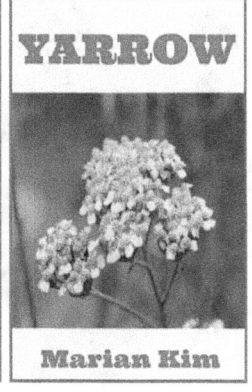

Marian Kim

*****

www.ingramcontent.com/pod-product-compliance
Lightning Source LLC
Chambersburg PA
CBHW071344310526
45790CB00018B/1359